Compassion

Caroline Latham is the author of four books and is currently writing her fifth. She has been a therapist, healer and coach for nearly three decades, both treating individuals from across the globe and running workshops internationally. Caroline has worked with a huge range of clients, has set up a charity (www.canterburytibetlink.org.uk) and has run mindfulness groups for over twenty years. Her 'Common Sense Therapy' accesses the root of clients' emotional blocks, and helps to alleviate suffering. Her aim is to benefit those she helps as much as possible.

Sheldon Mindfulness

A full list of titles is available from Sheldon Press,
36 Causton Street, London SW1P 4ST and on our website at
www.sheldonpress.co.uk

Sheldon Mindfulness

Compassion

CAROLINE LATHAM

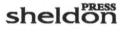

First published in Great Britain in 2015

Sheldon Press
36 Causton Street
London SW1P 4ST
www.sheldonpress.co.uk

A catalogue record for this book is available from the British Library

ISBN 978-1-84709-407-0
eBook ISBN 978-1-84709-408-7

Typeset by Fakenham Prepress Solutions, Fakenham, Norfolk NR21 8NN
First printed in Great Britain by Ashford Colour Press
Subsequently digitally reprinted in Great Britain

eBook by Fakenham Prepress Solutions, Fakenham, Norfolk NR21 8NN

Produced on paper from sustainable forests

Contents

Acknowledgements

This book would not have been conceived without the suggestion of my editor, Fiona Marshall, to whom I am deeply grateful.

But my deepest gratitude will always go to my teachers. I would have been on the scrapheap without their guidance, compassion and wisdom. I am so blessed. Jigme Khyentse Rinpoche, this is your copyright.

Gratitude too to Chuck Spezzano, whose words I repeatedly quote. He has told me he wants his work to carry on and I hope his methods will become increasingly widespread, because they work. Thank you for being so funny as well as great at emotional emergency kits!

Finally, gratitude to you, my readers. Know that buying a copy of this book will help many charitable projects and make more peace in the world. Ninety per cent of the book's profits are dedicated to <www.songtsen.org> (the Kangyur Rinpoche Foundation).

Thank you all!

Sheldon Mindfulness

Compassion

Introduction: Mindfulness and compassion

This book has one motivation: to be of benefit to all sentient beings. May it benefit you and everyone else, far and wide, as profoundly and as much as is possible!

My aim has been to write this book in the simplest possible way, because my editor and I really want it to be practical, easy to read and to the point. 'Simple can be harder than complex' is a Steve Jobs quotation I just happened to read . . . So let's simply keep it simple.

So what is the link between mindfulness and compassion? To be 'mindful' means to be aware. The opposite of mindfulness is being lost in mindless thinking or thoughtless actions. Compassion means being aware of another person's suffering with a deep desire to do something to relieve it. By practising mindfulness, we can develop enough attention to act in such a way as to help others by thinking and then behaving more compassionately.

Nobody has 'time' these days, so I've tried to be practical and succinct. I hope this will allow you to absorb what all this 'mindful compassion' is about easily and quickly and 'get to it' straight away. That is my wish. I'm not suggesting in any way that this is a quick fix. I would like to help set you on the path of training your mind in the most compassionate way in order to discover its true nature and its true power. It can take a lifetime to master the techniques included within these pages. But you can start where you are right now and stop where you're not.

I have been practising meditation, mindfulness and compassionate mind training for over a quarter of a century now, and have done some form of practice every day – except one. I clearly remember that particular day. It was not a good day.

Therefore I can vouch for the efficacy of these practices. I have been fortunate to be taught them by some of the best teachers in the world, people who are living and constant embodiments of compassion. I owe my teachers everything. All that is helpful in this book comes from them. Anything that is unhelpful comes from me.

I have also been fortunate to be able to pass these practices on to thousands of people from every background over several decades. Some have taken them up with alacrity, while many others have let them fall by the wayside, but it is fair to say that those who have kept them up report that their lives have been transformed and say how very much better they feel.

This is important.

There are benefits to these practices and they are evident. The greatest benefit is becoming calmer and feeling happier. Other benefits include lower blood pressure, greater longevity, fewer wrinkles, more energy, less need for sleep, greater efficiency and improved memory (although personally I haven't noticed that one yet).

In my capacity as a therapist and healer over a career spanning nearly 30 years, I have picked up a helpful trick or two. These can help when mindfulness or the ability to practise appears to be blocked. They are not the ultimate solution but they are an aid along the way. My aim in this book is to distil what I have learnt from my years of mind training and therapeutic practice into the most essential methods to help you to begin to train your mind in the techniques of mindful compassion.

Read this book. Try out all the exercises. Come back at the end of the year and let me know whether or not you have felt the benefit. If it has so much as turned you a thumbnail away from unhappiness, it is a thumbnail's worth in the right direction. As with anything, it requires effort. (Effort is not everyone's favourite word but it sounds much more appealing than discipline.) 'If at first you don't succeed, try and try again.'

Not that there is a 'success' to be achieved. The success I am talking about means letting go of the wish to be successful and accepting everything as being perfect as it is. Success, in this case, means freedom. It is true, though, that to be good at anything you have to keep at it. Perhaps this quotation is better: 'Do a little more than is easy and a little less than is hard.'

Please don't class yourself as one of those people who simply can't do it. 'Oh, I've tried that meditation stuff, and it's just not for me.' I've heard that a lot, but it can be just an excuse for you to stay stuck where you are. It's a bit like saying you won't like baked beans when you've just looked at the tin on the shelf in the supermarket. Or refusing to keep on taking the medicine when you've just swallowed one pill of a course of antibiotics because 'it's not working'. You don't know which bit is going to work, even though the doctor has told you how important it is to complete the course.

As long as you can breathe, you can practise mindful compassion.

You might not want to. You might want to pooh-pooh the evidence that it will do you good, but if you could see the inside of your mind you might reconsider. Just as looking at your protruding stomach might encourage you to start a diet, examining the quality, or lack of quality, of your thinking might encourage you to 'take yourself in hand'.

I often say to people that I would be on the scrapheap if I hadn't taken up meditation. I genuinely believe this to be true and would like to wish all of you out there to try out what is within these pages.

You might suffer from jumbled thinking, anxiety, depression or addiction; or you might be one of the few who isn't suffering at the moment, and yet you might admit that you could be happier or would like to help someone else who is suffering. If either or both the above are your current position, please have a go, and make a real effort to stick with the meditation practices within these pages for at least 12 months.

Compassion works. It makes you happier. And it makes others happier too.

Part 1

The blocks

Part 1.

The blacks

1

Refuge beyond neurosis

If you have picked up this book, there is a good chance that you would like to learn about mindfulness and compassion. It may be, of course, that somebody bought the book for you. In which case, nothing happens by accident, so I hope you won't ignore their kind suggestion.

Mindfulness is very fashionable at the moment, but there is a reason for its being so successful: contrary to the former notion that it is only for hippies, now it is becoming de rigueur in most circles. Why? Because it works. Because advances in science mean we are better able to weigh and measure its efficacy.

Efficacy at what?

It is pretty clear, whether we like it or not, that at some point in our lives we have all felt pain. Even little children become sick or lose their favourite toy or get upset because their mother tells them off, while many of us suffer from what we might call major problems, such as starvation and earthquakes. The bottom line is that we all feel pain at some point, and it is inescapable.

Mindfulness is a tried and tested method of training our mind to cope with that pain and even to go beyond it.

If someone were to hit us repeatedly with a stick, we would eventually learn that, if we could, moving out of the way might be helpful. It is we who take the action of moving out of the way. The important thing is how we deal with the situation.

If we were in prison, whether guilty or not guilty, it would be the way we coped with the situation that would bring us relief or otherwise. We would not, in general, be able to escape. We would need to use our mind to cope.

If we are suffering because we are in a tricky situation, we might not be able to change the outer circumstances, but surely we can change our attitude towards them. It may not stop the situation occurring or make it disappear, but it could enable us to handle it better.

Clinging to a problem makes us stick to the past, the block, and to stay stuck in the unhappy, troublesome or nightmarish event instead of letting go and trusting a refuge.

Trusting a refuge in this sense simply means that there is a place beyond where our thinking is stuck, caught in its ratchet of repetitive neurosis. I do not mean to start this book by insulting you all, but that repetitive thinking, that ratchet is called **neurotic thought**. And in that sense we all suffer from neurosis.

Beginning to realize that we are all caught in this neurotic thinking, or what is often called 'monkey mind', is the beginning of developing awareness. It is the beginning of minding the gap. We begin to take note of the gap between our neurotic thinking and our awareness of it flitting about this way and that.

Worrying about the future means taking up time worrying about something that might never happen. There is a marvellous Tibetan saying: 'Why worry? If something's going to happen, it will happen anyway, so what's the point in worrying about it? And if it's not going to happen, what's the point in worrying about it?'

If we broke a leg, we would trust the ambulance to take us to a hospital. We would trust that the hospital would have a doctor capable of setting the leg properly. We would trust the refuge of the hospital and the treatment. We would trust that, thanks to the treatment, we would eventually be able to walk again without pain.

Very few of us would stay at home alone, nursing the break and the agony. Most likely, going to hospital and finding refuge in a doctor and treatment would mean that a day would come when we would no longer even think about the broken leg.

Refuge means there is always a safe space. It means there is a space in our mind beyond the neurotic monkey mind. There is a place that is always free and clear and pure and without the burden of restricted vision. Letting go is safe. Refuge is foolproof. It never lets you down. It never runs out on you. It is the state of as-it-is-ness.

Men, women, family, friends, things, drugs, hobbies may at some point let you down. Therefore finding refuge in the truth of your mind beyond its neurotic thinking patterns can be a huge, reliable and true support. It is worth investigating what I am saying here because it is through your own personal experience that you will know it to be true. Anyone can tell you anything, but it is your experience that counts. Test it out. Investigate it. Read more research, but examine your own mind most of all. Try it out. It's worth a try.

The process can lead you from mindlessness to mindfulness.

Mindfulness can be defined as *awareness of thoughts, feelings, sensations and the surrounding environment now, in this moment*, and acceptance thereof. It is an awareness of thoughts and feelings *without judging whether they are right or wrong*.

It means peace.

It's about calming down more and more.

Exercise 1

Put your phone down and hide it away for three minutes.

Close the door.

Lock the bathroom door if need be for a bit of peace, even if you are at work.

Breathe.

Breathe in, push your stomach out.

Breathe out, pull your stomach in.

Breathe in and out through your nose if you can. Put your hands on your stomach if you find that helpful.

Imagine you are filling up the balloon of your stomach as you breathe in and emptying the balloon of your stomach as you breathe out.

If it helps, imagine a line going from your nose, through your throat, down through your lungs and into your stomach and another line going back up from your stomach, up and out through your nose. (Don't complicate things if you don't need to visualize that.)

You don't need to think of anything special. You can if you wish but otherwise, simply breathe.

Breathe, you are alive.

Caution: do not do this more than three times in one go. It is not about hyperventilating. It is simply about taking the time for three conscious breaths. That's all.

Exercise 1a

Even simpler:

Just breathe, and notice you're breathing.

_____

2

Interdependence

It seems that nowadays even children at school learn that interdependence is the way of things. Interdependence means that everything is connected. Conversely, it means nothing exists independently. Everything exists in relation to something else.

In the natural world, no organism is cut off from its surroundings. Organisms are a part of their environment, which is rich in living and non-living elements that interact in various ways. The interactions of an organism with its environment are vital to its survival and to the functioning of the ecosystem as a whole.

You think you are alone, you think your thoughts are independent, but actually you are connected to the air you breathe, the trees that produce the oxygen, the bees, the birds, etc.

A very old friend and teacher of mine, the psychologist Chuck Spezzano, once said: 'There's no such thing as a private thought.' It scared the living daylights out of me.

Then there is chaos theory, often expressed in simple form as the 'butterfly effect'. This is a mathematical model explaining the way in which tiny events such as a butterfly flapping its wings can have massive effects such as creating a hurricane on the other side of the world. It's an extreme example, but it does show up how crucially interconnected everything is.

The bad news is that this means everything you do affects someone or something else. It means that others are constantly affecting you. Less disturbingly, the good news is that it means you can never be truly alone.

What has this got to do with mindful compassion? Everything.

If you cannot act completely alone, you may act differently. If you realize that your action has consequences that affect others, you may act differently.

If you know you are never truly alone, you may act less independently and ask for help more often. You may then act differently.

You only have to watch television to see that nowadays an incident in India, the USA, China or any other country can be broadcast across the world in less than a few minutes, affecting world politics. Even the most distant regions are no longer remote.

The reason for mentioning this is the importance of truly understanding it. It is more than a concept. When my old schoolfriend Barbara put a very brief sentence up on Facebook, 'I am getting married', within seconds she was bombarded with congratulations from across the globe and was extremely embarrassed to have to admit that the statement of her impending marriage had been a joke. Or the Twitter nightmare when someone reads your 15 words and misunderstands them and you have to deal with unpleasant feedback and cyber-bullying, and perhaps with adverse consequences in your home, work or school life.

I often describe each one of us as a piece of a puzzle, but an important one. We might have knobbly bits or bits that stick out, or we might be a bit bent, but we are all necessary and all part of the whole puzzle. Even if we are missing, we are still part of the puzzle!

So if you truly understand that we are all one, that we are all interconnected, you will know that acting helpfully and with awareness will lead others to benefit. You simply cannot act in isolation and expect your helpful action to lead to a helpful reaction. To quote John Donne, 'No man is an island.'

If you want external disarmament, start with internal disarmament.

Exercise 2

Wherever you are, whatever you are doing, stop for a few minutes. Even just one minute. Just 60 seconds.

If you are happy, say silently to yourself:
'May my happiness go out and benefit all those who aren't so happy.'

If you are unhappy, say silently to yourself:
'May my unhappiness alleviate the unhappiness everyone else is going through.'

That's it.

Very simple.

Just do it! That's the key. It's all about bothering to take those few seconds out and do it. In those few seconds you can help so many others and help yourself.

It's worth a try. It's worth a few tries. It could well be worth a lifetime of tries. It's certainly better than being stuck in your own misery or being guilty or big-headed about your happiness.

It serves a useful purpose.

3

Why compassion?

Rarely do we think about what the word compassion really means. We tend to use it more in a negative or complaining fashion, for example, 'Well, they could have showed more compassion, couldn't they?'

Or we might describe someone as 'very compassionate', by which we mean very kind. We may have a sense that someone has been born with a compassionate nature and is therefore always going to be compassionate. It is true that some people appear so, but this makes the idea of compassion passive – in fact compassion can be very active.

It helps to realize that the brain can be trained. It's now increasingly recognized that the brain can reorganize its neural pathways in response to experience or sensory stimulation – a capability known as **brain plasticity** – and our understanding of this is replacing beliefs held until recently that the brain was pretty much 'stuck in place'. Thus we have an important role to play in bringing about changes to our brain and then living with those changes.

Dr Susan Taylor, a nutritional biochemist who has studied yogic sciences for over 30 years, says:

> Positive thoughts expand our brains. Negative thoughts shrink them. The brain has neuroplasticity – it can change and be moulded like plastic. The biggest factors creating these changes are our thoughts and emotions. 'Self-directed neuroplasticity' means consciously influencing our minds in positive ways, such as meditation, that expand our brains and enable us to receive what we need to lead a fulfilling and happy life.

This means we can control our minds a lot more than we thought we could. And it is how we apply the control that is the interesting question. The idea that we can actually train our mind to develop more compassion can be seen as something frightfully novel, or something to which we feel resistance. Why not just train our mind to improve our memory, to improve our general knowledge or to obtain the highest IQ? Why train our mind to develop compassion? Why not just stick with mindfulness and learn how to relax a bit more?

But where will simply learning to relax a bit more or improving our memory lead? These are certainly short-term benefits, and marvellous ones, of course. Equally, however, I have heard people say that mindfulness is being used to train soldiers to improve their aim when shooting . . . Mindfulness could inadvertently become a minefield. (Forgive the dreadful pun!)

Yet we could go further . . .

Let us look at the definition of compassion. According to the etymological definition, compassion means to 'suffer with'. Hardly a sales point. The most common understanding of the word, meanwhile, is 'to empathize' or 'to feel with'. So how on earth can compassion be something one would voluntarily wish to do?

I'm sure many of you have been brought up to be kind, to do your duty, to respect and help others. But compassion? Have you spent time thinking about compassion or how it might improve the quality of your life? Most likely for many of you, your reaction would be, 'What's that all about?' It's not something we often talk about or consider.

I hope those who have already spent a lifetime developing more compassion will forgive me. What follows is for those who haven't.

For those of you who don't know, the facts are simple. Compassion helps you. Compassion is the most selfish thing you can do, because you yourself benefit.

It is satisfying to live in an age when doubters can have their doubts dissolved. Science is our twentieth- and twenty-first-century god. And according to science, developing compassion increases our happiness.

Most often we think ourselves to be very important and our basic desire is to help ourselves to be happy and ensure that things to go well for us. Yet we don't know how to bring these things about. Actually, such a self-cherishing attitude makes us very uptight. In fact, acting out of a self-cherishing attitude can never make us happy.

Mindfulness is important in that it enables us to become aware of when we are doing things that are harmful to ourselves and to others, but compassion is the key transforming agent of the mind.

There are different levels to compassion. At its simplest, it is a wish to be kind and helpful to others and to ourselves. At a deeper level it is connected to wisdom.

To understand the ideas above fully, and truly to understand the value of compassion, would require us to apply mindfulness and compassion exercises for many years. But we do get glimpses of what it is all about: that which could be described as beyond matter and awareness; that which is truly important and makes us what we really are. Those glimpses can sustain us when we slip into a trough of laziness.

But it is not just experience that proves the validity of developing compassion. It has been shown in tests, as detailed in Matthieu Ricard's book, *Happiness* (Little, Brown, 2006):

> As they began meditating on compassion, an extraordinary increase of left prefrontal activity was registered. Compassion, the very act of feeling concern for other people's well-being, appears to be one of the positive emotions, like joy and enthusiasm. This corroborates the research of psychologists showing that the most altruistic members of a population are also those who enjoy the highest sense of satisfaction in life . . . Lutz, Davidson and their colleagues also found that the brain activity of the practitioners meditating on compassion was especially high in the left prefrontal cortex. Activity in the left prefrontal cortex swamped activity in the right prefrontal (site of negative emotions and anxiety), something never before seen from purely mental activity . . .

Or, quoting from Paul Gilbert in *Mindful Compassion* (Robinson, 2013):

> What our attention focuses on will stimulate very different brain systems and emotions. It is not our fault our minds get pulled away from the present moment in the ways they do. This is to do with the evolution of our 'new brain' capacities and how our minds have developed from our life experiences. It is important to frame mindfulness training within a compassionate orientation. When unaddressed issues begin to surface, such as feelings of grief, shame, self-criticism or self-loathing, compassion enables us to hold these feelings with kindness and understanding. Mindfulness heals wounds and offers a sense of connectedness.

Responsibility for our world doesn't just depend on our leaders. It depends on each of us individually. Peace starts within each one of us. When we have inner peace, we can be at peace with those around us. The practice of mindfulness leads to greater calm, and that state of calm allows us to understand the value of developing more compassion.

Reflecting on the fact that everything is interdependent helps us to understand that other is actually a part of ourselves. Understanding this is critical if we are to get the point. To return to what I said in the last chapter, if we do not exist independently and solidly and uniquely, then it follows that others are part of us.

Where were you when 9/11 happened, or the Asian tsunami, or the earthquake in Nepal? I challenge any of you to deny feeling affected. Did you then just try and switch off? Did you cry? What use were those tears other than to show you aren't a hard cynical brute?

In an essay in the *Boston Review*, Yale psychologist Paul Bloom takes unlikely aim at empathy. He attacks empathy not because it's impossible to feel other people's pain – he thinks we can, in fact, experience the plight of another person – but because such a state of mind does a disservice to both the empathizer and the individual on the receiving end and fails to make the world a better place.

People in pain don't want you to feel their pain; they want you to be there for them.

The exciting news is that practising compassion can actually help with those situations, both close to home and far away. Your thinking can change the world.

> Commit yourself to a daily practice,
> your loyalty to that is like a ring on the door.
> Keep knocking and eventually the joy that lives inside
> will look out to see who's there . . .
>
> Rumi (thirteenth-century Persian poet and Sufi mystic)

I would like to include a true anecdote here. I worked in a clinic for several years. There was a guy who worked there who was known as the 'secret angel'. He helped people others couldn't reach. One day, we actually had time for a brief chat.

He asked me: 'Do you remember a beggar who was grouchy and bad tempered and used to sit on a dirty blanket with his two wild dogs? He sat on the pavement in the High Street. He was always grumbling and he always had a bottle in his hand.'

I told him I did. He was there for a very long time and my children got used to giving him money as they passed by. He had looked dirty and grimy and distinctly angry and troubled.

'That beggar was me,' the counsellor said.

I was flabbergasted. In front of me was a quiet and respectable chap in clean clothes and with a gentle temperament.

One day he reached the conclusion that he had had enough of his current life and decided to sober up. He cleaned himself up, got a job and saved. He then walked three times around the sacred Mount Kailash in Tibet, an act which he had been told would purify the error of his previous ways – even though he was born an Irish Catholic and no longer belonged to any particular faith. He returned to the UK and has since become very compassionate and sober. He's settled down and has a growing family now.

If he can, you can.

Exercise 3: Give to all who ask

This exercise involves moving. If you can't, don't worry. Simply imagine yourself doing it.

Today, give to all who ask.

You know, the beggar you always walk past because you think he should get a job. Or the busker whose music you loathe – and anyway, you're in too much of a hurry to reach into your pocket. Or the child who wants more pocket money. Or don't refuse when your partner asks you to collect the children when you were planning to watch some gripping match or other programme on television. Whatever you usually avoid or miss or ignore.

Take the trouble.

If you can't give to all who ask, at least give a little to more people than you usually do.

Exercise 3a

If you found the previous exercise too hard, try this one:

Just put a penny in your right hand and offer it to your left hand – or imagine doing so. Offer the penny to your left hand with kindness and generosity.

That's it. That simple action can break the tightness of 'being stuck'.

4

Tap into your good heart

What would be your first instinct if you saw a child being run over in the street as you were walking by?

For several decades I have asked each and every client I see what he or she would do in this situation. They all, without fail, each and every one of them, have said they would want to help. That means that even if at a conscious level you might feel blocked or resistant, at an unconscious level your primordial wish is to help. Ergo, you have a good heart. Otherwise, would not at least one client have said, 'Exterminate! Exterminate!'?

But not a single one ever has. And I have seen some very tricky people.

The theory is that only 6 per cent of you is conscious, if that. By calling in help from your unconscious mind, you are accessing a part of you that is infinitely more powerful than your conscious self. But you need to ask for help. Otherwise, how can the help get in?

Connecting with your unconscious mind leads you beyond the ratchet zone, the zone of neurotic thought. It reconnects you to the 'sky-like nature of your mind'. It helps you to remember the sky, or calm, beyond your neurotic thinking.

In Tibet the word 'blessing' can be translated as 'the sound of waves in your ears'. In other words you need to know the sound is there, let the waves transmit the sound and have your ears open to let the sound in. Once again, it's all about 'connecting' to the inter-dependent state of all of us.

The more you become aware of not buying into neurotic chatter and letting it lead you wherever it wants, the more you can begin to access your compassionate mind.

I have witnessed thousands of people call in help in the way I describe here and at least a hundred, no doubt more, have found tears springing up in their eyes. This is nothing to do with magic. It is to do with connecting with your own good heart and it can be hugely comforting. It might not be as strong as diving into a mother's bosom as a baby, but it can be a good second best and it only depends on you doing it.

There really is no getting away from the fact that it is your choice. To do or not to do. To call in help or not to call in help.

But how?

Easy. Here goes.

Exercise 4: Calling in help

Take in three deep breaths.

  Breathe in, push your stomach out.

  Breathe out, pull your stomach in.

  Let go.

  Now that you are a little calmer, think of your good heart. If you have a particular faith, call on God, call on Buddha, or call on Allah. Call on all of them; call on your 'high power', the universe, Gaia, the scientific state of interdependence, whatever you want to call it.

  If none of those suit, call on the power of your good heart. You know your good heart is there, even if it has gone underground.

  Say something like: 'God help me!'

  You probably say that anyway even if you're a confirmed atheist. Funny how we do that.

  If that idea makes you uncomfortable, try something like:

  'Good heart' – whatever you want to call it – 'that stuff beyond my conscious mind, please help!'

  Or simply: 'HELP!'

  If you're still perplexed, do what I recommend to children: call in 'the force'.

Don't just pay lip service to this. Do it truly. It's free, and it's your life we're talking about.

The effect is instantaneous.

Remember that I have seen very tough people reduced to tears through this simple action. So trust your own power. Nobody other than you is doing anything. But doing it and trusting its effect is key.

That's it.

Do it whenever you think about it. Preferably thousands of times a day.

5

Why some of us become addicted to negative emotions

What I wrote in the previous chapter has probably made some of you want to throw this book down in fury. (Note the anger indicated by the word 'fury'.) I do so hope you haven't. Compassion is exciting.

The point is that we often prefer to stay blind, not realizing that there is a zone in which we can be so much happier than we have been until now. Nelson Mandela always used to quote the words of Marianne Williamson: 'Our deepest fear is not that we are inadequate. Our deepest fear is that we are powerful beyond measure.'

That is because that zone is unfamiliar to us. We tend to limit ourselves to what we know. We are afraid of happiness. Yes, we are afraid of experiencing more happiness than we are used to.

If we have smoked all our lives, we become afraid of stopping smoking. We think we will be unhappy if we stop and without realizing it, we lie to ourselves, ignoring the evidence that we would be happier, wealthier and healthier.

The same applies to all habits and all addictions. We become addicted to the habit or the addiction. We think that the bottle, the bet, the sex, the drug, the cigarette, or even the cup of tea is what makes us happy, so why should we stop? What guarantee do we have that more happiness will be the result?

The same applies to all negative emotions. Some people might have a habit or addiction to some negative emotion. For example:

- Are you afraid of something and maybe scared to take action to conquer that fear?
- Are you often or habitually angry without taking steps to quell that anger?
- Are you full of envy, yet find it hard to let go of the 'grass is greener' syndrome?
- Have you ever obsessed about a would-be lover?

Yet happiness comes from doing the opposite of these things.

We often aren't aware of that fact and we certainly don't want to trust it. It is similar to an animal in captivity beginning to think that its plight is the norm. It is similar to a person who has worked all her life finding when she retires that she doesn't know what to do. Yet all her life she has dreamt of the day when she will be able to retire and not have to get up to go to work.

Being free of any type of niggling habit or addiction means being truly happy, and being truly happy does indeed frighten us. Yet, as my teacher Jigme Khyentse Rinpoche said: 'If you were being chased by guerrillas with guns and an aeroplane were taking off allowing you to get away free, would you run towards freedom or hang around and get shot?'

Many of us just don't seem to understand that maintaining our habits of going to the shop to buy our cigarettes or bottle of wine, placing our bet, watching our favourite soap, eating our chocolate biscuit, or even ringing a family member or friend, doesn't give us the happiness we really want. One gambler confided in me that even when his debts were cleared and he had no further need of it, he had to go out and borrow more money because he couldn't 'live without a loan'. It made him feel too uncomfortable.

Think about what might happen if we got out of those negative habits of mind, our clinging and negative emotions.

- Where would we be if we stopped moaning about what others have and we don't?
- Where would we be if we stopped getting an adrenalin high out of losing our temper?
- Where would we be if we stopped obsessing about a dream partner who may well not be available? We might actually fall in love . . .
- Where would we be if we minded that gap and let something different and better come in?

Does such a life frighten you and send you straight back to 'using'?

If so, join the majority of us who are dealing with the same conundrum. These addictions start with our mind. It is not the bottle flying off the shelf into our lap or the cork popping out of its own accord. It is not our tone of voice rising of its own accord. It is our mind that encourages the vocal cords. It is our clinging to the notion that the contents of our mind will give us what we seek. It is our clinging to the thought.

The Mind and Life Institute runs conferences with luminaries every year and recently covered the topic of addiction. It showed how the issue starts with desire.

Now the same mind can be turned to desiring either in a positive way or a negative way. If left uncontrolled, negative desire leads to craving, and then it can worsen and lead to addiction. Training our brain to redirect our desire is the solution.

But it is, as always, up to us. Nobody can do it for us. If it could be done for us, it would lead to a world of lobotomized robots and we as individuals would be no happier. Therefore we are back where we started.

Yes, it takes effort to train our mind. But not training our mind can lead to unfortunate consequences. If we train our mind out of its addictions we develop a sense of freedom and develop power. We develop the power to choose. With that choice we could choose something we know would make us happier. That is the way of compassion. That compassion could then benefit others as well as ourselves.

I can, hand on heart, assure you that people who do bother to train their minds out of unhelpful addictions and obsessions, those who meditate and train in compassion, lead much happier and more fulfilling lives. Many have 'fallen' or come down from what society calls great heights, but beyond the so-called fall, these people have found themselves, their hearts and their life.

An ex-heroin addict friend of mine called Big Oliver puts it most succinctly (and he oozes compassion): 'Just place your mind elsewhere.'

Exercise 5

Try and notice at least once today when your mind is thinking poisonous thoughts. Change them. Apply the antidote. Put in an opposite positive thought.

For example, when someone offends you, don't go spinning off into, 'How dare they?' – and spend ten minutes or ten days being offended and keeping the conversation going in your head.

Every time you catch yourself thinking, 'How could he have said or done that to me, after all I've done for him?' simply say to yourself silently:

'Thank you.'

The other person wins if you carry on the negative thinking. By saying thank you, you win, because you are free. You can even be grateful because that person has given you the opportunity to clear your negative, jumbled thinking and become aware of *now*, which is hugely positive. You can't change what they've said or done but you can let go and make space for the truth in the now.

You can choose to be compassionate *now*.

You can feel gratitude because without that person you would not have had to become aware of your thoughts and take responsibility for changing them.

Exercise 5b

Let's get down to basics.

When your usual rush hour train is cancelled and you are left waiting for three hours, having to stand because your local station no longer provides any seats, breathe and come into the present. Don't do what you might normally do by making it personal and thinking it is only you going through the discomfort. Try and remember that others around you are in the same situation. Don't scream. Don't go into it. Try and gain a sense of spaciousness.

Pretend you are a saint and try to see it all as a dream. Say to yourself:

'I want to be the Dalai Lama. I want to be Mother Teresa.'

Go on, have a go.

Exercise 5c

If someone around you is failing you and you are complaining about it, think instead about how you can support that person.

Exercise 5d

Forgive whoever it is you are blaming, because in forgiving others you are forgiving yourself for some past event. Then join that person in your mind or your heart with love and honest communication.

However tricky it is to do this, not to do so means you stay in the hurt and perpetuate the problem within your family and your relationships. Is it not worth it to live more happily and fully?

Exercise 5e

At the root of all problems is fear. There is either love or fear.

When fear is blocking you from joining your 'enemy', the 'other person', visualize the block as a wall between yourself and that person.

Call in help and dissolve the wall with whatever machinery you wish to create.

Don't cheat. Demolish the wall completely. Don't simply make enough space to climb over or break through – tear it all down.

Only stop when the wall is completely dissolved and only dust remains.

Imagine stepping through and hugging the other person.

6

Blocks to compassion

Wouldn't we all like to avoid hurting and being hurt if we could? There are people who do manage to do this. Their brains are so finely tuned as to stay beyond the ratchet of neurotic thinking. They appear to be calm at all times. But many of us can't avoid feeling and causing pain, as I have already explained, because we are so often helplessly caught in that ratchet.

This neurotic thinking pattern can be examined and explained theoretically and scientifically through MRI scans which can show the effect of meditation on the brain. Neurotic thinking of this kind can often form blocks to compassion. These blocks, which can prevent us from even wanting to consider developing compassion, may well have developed in early childhood.

Sadly, many of us experience very early on in life some lack of self-worth or a sense of lacking love, and this may stop us loving or accepting ourselves fully. We might not consciously use that kind of language, or even be consciously aware of it, but the effect is that we get used to 'putting up with' less than we deserve, and consequently offering less of it around.

We suffer so much from this lack of self-love, especially in the West. If a lack of self-love is the norm, it follows that it becomes difficult to step out into the unknown because we don't know what it means to do so. If we always wear dark glasses, taking them off will make us feel odd and the world seem strange, even if the view is better and brighter.

Many people seem to think they've got to go out and 'get' something to be loveable instead of realizing it is within them already.

How can the love get in if your heart isn't open? How can it get out?

It is important to realize that it is our blocks that are stopping the love getting either in or out. We can be so busy working that, however much someone is trying to love us, it is impossible because they never see us. And if we are conked out on the sofa having overindulged, it is impossible for us to reach out to someone or for someone to reach in. Any excuse. Why?

Because somewhere along the line we have been so badly hurt that we put up a barrier. We put up an invisible sign saying 'Keep out'. And it limits us. It is none other than pride. This might not be the definition you are used to, but it is what sets us up to feel either better or worse than someone else. It makes us feel special. It is what separates us from the true state of interdependence.

Imagine a drawing in which your thinking is represented by a dot. The more you think, the more the dot grows, thicker and deeper and bigger. It is simply the 'you that thinks'.

But the mind doesn't stop at one thought. It continues to turn around and mull over a succession of thoughts. The thoughts seem very solid and real.

These thoughts make you feel separate, but we know already that your thoughts do not exist independently as you imagined. Nor are they permanent. Soon the thoughts will pass, however obsessed you are and however much you think they won't. However, because of your pain, because of your habit, because of the way you've been brought up, you prefer to think of your thoughts, feelings and perceptions as being you – and as being a separate and independent 'you'.

That is pride. Pride separates and pride hurts. *If it hurts, it's pride.*

Truth does not hurt. When someone says something hurtful to you and you bridle, it's because of that sense of self. It's where you've erected that wall against the world. If you could, you'd like to hide behind that wall and stay there.

Fundamentally, *isn't it annoying that there is the 'other'!!!*

The belief in and emphasis on that dot of thought is what creates the pain. Yet you think protecting yourself from what is 'other' will stop the pain. Not so. Believing that thought to be solid and independent hurts more. It can lead to a strong sense of independence and wanting always to 'go it alone'; it can even, in my humble opinion, lead at its worst extreme to psychosis.

Compassion is the realization that 'it' does not exist solidly and independently for either you or the other. There are no barriers. There is no separation. Compassion is the wish for others to understand that too.

Exercise 6

Make the firm resolution now to be free of your neurotic thinking.

When you 'stick' to negative thoughts and actions again and again, the pain is continually reinforced.

Decide and make a strong wish to start checking what is on/in your mind and choose whether you want to feel better or worse. Put in its bluntest form, do you want to go in a life direction or a death direction?

Resolve again and again to be happy. And why not, at the same time, add all the seven other billion people on the planet?

May all beings be happy and free from pain.

It's that simple a thought. And thoughts are very powerful.

If you feel resistance to doing this, remember when you were last really happy. Savour the feelings. Do you want that or what you are feeling now? It's your choice.

And again. Do you want to be 'right' or do you want to be happy?

7

Guilt

To recap, developing compassion leads to a state of freedom in which we do not cling to our neurotic thinking and way of seeing. We are free and therefore happier and have increasing compassion for others.

However, such a state is rare. I know of one family where there was never a raised voice in the household, although it contained six children. Nothing but love was expressed. That is the only family I have ever heard declare this as being the truth. It's a rarity. The rest of us have to make do with the best our parents can manage. Show me one parent on the planet who could put their hand up and say their parenting had been perfect.

We all make mistakes. The issue is that we like to stick to the mistake, or prefer to indulge in guilt and self-hatred – many older people will resonate with the words *mea culpa, mea culpa* ('my fault, my fault').

Self-blame serves to maintain our neurotic thinking. It serves to keep us in pain. It gives us the excuse to berate ourselves and then carry on indulging the mistake.

Here's an example. I recently played tennis with someone and was aware of playing badly, but so was my partner. Both of us felt deeply embarrassed about missing so many easy shots, but the act of feeling embarrassed persisted in keeping the concentration and focus on ourselves and the embarrassment itself rather than allowing us to move on. We reinforced the mistakes every time we said, 'Sorry, sorry, sorry.' If we had moved on and concentrated on the present moment instead of harping on about the missed serve or the stupid mistake, we would have played much better.

In the case of addiction, it gives us the excuse to carry on drinking or using.

'I'm such a bad person, I can't face what I have/haven't done.' So the only thing to do is to hide, by maintaining or increasing the addiction . . . But we all know that hiding doesn't work; it just exacerbates the problem, emphasizing the selfishness and focus on oneself. It means going ever further underground into one's ego. But we can't blot out the ego, however many bottles we down.

One client of mine complained of the times when her ex-husband came to parents' meetings. They would both sit there purportedly to hear what the teacher had to say about their son. But she was sad to report that her ex-husband was more intent on telling the teacher how guilty he felt for not being at home any more and not helping with the homework. The son looked on, bemused and dismayed. The teacher didn't get a word in edgeways to talk about how the son was actually doing. So intent was the father on saying how guilty he felt, he had no chance of getting on with living the present situation.

Guilt is the superglue of the ego and locks into your negative thinking instead of finding the error, correcting it and moving forward. It is a Western speciality. There is no word for guilt in Tibetan! There is only one word for revenge in Tibetan and many for compassion.

We all indulge in guilt, and it pops up, like a tenacious weed, when you thought you had cleared it.

Chuck Spezzano, whom I mentioned earlier, has written many books, and I couldn't help laughing when I noticed that his book on guilt was one of his thickest! To quote him, 'There are no bad guys – not even you.'

It might be helpful to mention that everyone tends to feel guilt when someone dies. We always wish we had seen them that one last time, said that one last thing or not left the room at the critical moment. Yet it is well documented that some people appear to choose to die when they are alone, rather than when their relatives or friends are present. Hospice workers describe how a person may appear to wait until everyone has left, even for a brief time, before taking his final breath. When I worked with the dying, I understood that it was because the relatives' grief can draw the dying person's consciousness back, which is not helpful.

Guilt is the most useless emotion, one that serves no useful purpose.
So here comes resolution.

Exercise 7: Transforming words

Every time you find yourself saying or thinking:
I should
I shouldn't
I ought
I oughtn't
I must
I mustn't

replace with:

'I choose'.

Exercise 7a

Every time you find yourself wandering around muttering: 'You stupid idiot, why oh why did I do that?' stop and correct yourself.

Say instead: 'I love and forgive myself.' Even if that kind of language feels alien and too sweet.

Go against that cynical you.

Give your arms a comforting pat.

Exercise 7b

Here is a serious exercise I have been taught which will help to resolve guilt.

When you've done something you feel bad about:
Call in that unconscious force for good – your good heart, or what-

ever else you would like to call it – whatever it is that you trust will help you more than the 6 per cent of your mind that is conscious.

Apologize for your unhelpful action.

Vow never to commit it again.

Ask for forgiveness.

And then forgive yourself.

Coat yourself in rainbow white light, as I describe in further detail in Chapter 14.

Make the light the consistency of a rainbow but the brightness of a full moon, and make sure you really do it.

Don't cheat on yourself and pretend you're doing it. Really do it. Pour the white light over yourself until you feel purified.

Then, when you've done it, let go.

What is gone is gone. What hasn't happened, hasn't happened yet.

Be in the now and trust.

8

From depression to compassion

We're still dealing with the reasons why we choose not to get out of our rut, why we choose not to develop compassion and be happy. It's worth reiterating that, because it reflects how our minds prefer to ruminate and dither and doubt. Somebody once said, 'Doubt is intelligence gone wrong.'

I used to run workshops where I asked the participants to sit opposite someone and spend ten minutes telling the other person their own qualities. After barely two or three minutes, most people dried up. I then asked them to spend ten minutes telling the listener their faults. Nobody ever ran out, gabbling away at a high level of intensity. Ten minutes was never enough.

This again is a particularly Western predilection, but one that, with globalization, seems to be increasingly affecting the East. Rates of depression in Japan, for example, are close to those in the West.

Winston Churchill called his depression his 'black dog', but I think the image of a huge black cloud is more appealing. Why? Because that is what it is. A black cloud. It is a state, and a state can change. As does everything.

Once again, the mind rushes to assume that it cannot change, that it is stuck forever in the prison of negative thinking. This is not possible, in the sense that everything is constantly changing. The good news is that depression will eventually pass, as huge black clouds do. The bad news is that the sun can seem to disappear too, and our happiness go underground. That is why we need to take refuge in knowing there is a state beyond the clouds; a state that is sky-like in its nature.

It's essential to remember this. The sky-like nature of our mind is always there, even when we can't access it.

It is important to write about depression, and even suicidal thoughts, because we need to acknowledge the sense of hopelessness it engenders. Depression is self-hatred, and suicide is the ultimate self-hatred; compassion on the other hand is the ultimate self-love. Depression makes us feel hopeless and stuck, and renders family members, friends or carers hopeless at helping too.

The thing is that we always want to run. Run towards happiness or run away from depression. But . . . There is always a 'but'! If we are stuck in bed because we are having a 'duvet-dive' day, we still cannot run from our thoughts. We might be avoiding work or avoiding 'life' but we are still stuck in our mind. Stuck in the repetitive configuration of neurotic thinking that makes us feel so hopeless. 'I want to die. I want to die. I can't live like this. I can't go on. I'm such a bad person. I'm so hopeless. I've screwed up so badly. I'm so unloveable. I'm so selfish.' And so on.

Where is the escape in that? Where is the escape when you are trapped in the prison of your own thoughts? If you spend long enough in this zone, you might reach this point: *The wisdom of no escape.*

So why no escape?

Because there is no proof that life does not exist after death, just as there is no proof to the contrary. Dr Sam Parnia, who has done research at Southampton University and the State University of New York, states: 'The evidence thus far suggests that in the first few minutes after death, consciousness is not annihilated.'

So if there is a possibility of life or consciousness after death, and there is so much anecdotal evidence of there being such a thing, then it is worth realizing that changing your mind in this life might be more effective while you still have the option to do so.

If it is possible that life does not end at death, then it is a high-risk strategy to imagine it will definitely do so. It is perhaps dangerous to gamble that after death will automatically be better. It may be much worse.

My personal understanding is that you are likely to take the way you are thinking at death with you. So it's best to take with you a positive train of thought, or at least to practise in order to take such a thing.

Getting out of that state of being 'stuck' is compassion towards yourself. Committing suicide therefore could be considered the most heinous act one could do to oneself.

Yes, depression can involve medication, but with the right medication and the right therapy (and the right therapist) – and affording the cost of treatment is compassion towards yourself too – then slowly but surely, you can train your mind out of its negative state of being stuck.

It is definitely worth the investment, because *you* are definitely worth the investment. In this interdependent world, you matter as much as any other person. You are no better or worse than the other, but you are equal and have equal value. *You are valuable.*

Count yourself in rather than out and have patience with yourself. Since you can't avoid your negative thoughts, try and make friends with them. Don't try and squash them like squashing a balloon: the un-squashed side tends to pop up even more when you do.

Exercise 8: Think of the other

When you are feeling your worst and completely stuck, think of someone who is worse off than you. You might pretend or feel that you are worse off than anyone else, but in fact there is always someone worse off than you are. Think of that one person. If you prefer, because you can't think of anyone, think of an animal. Focus on the person or animal.

Say to yourself:

'May my depression and my death wish take away theirs. May my pain alleviate theirs. May they feel better and live.'

That's it.

Every time you are stuck, think this.

Again and again.

And again.

If you think you can't, or find it hard to even finish the sentence, persist. Get out of your head and make that effort.

And if you wish, or can, maybe force yourself a little to add:

'Everything is constantly changing.'

One day it will sink in. It might be today or in the future, but it is definitely and absolutely worth doing. There are some states of mind so hellish that it is hard to even think of them. Places where you freeze and can never ever stop your teeth chattering; places where you burn and before you heal you burn again; places where you are eaten alive. We've all had those dreams or seen the films, or witnessed the lobsters being boiled alive.

Helping a person, or even an animal, out of those states is no waste of time. And it will help you out too.

Exercise 8a

Make sure you are taking care of your body as well as your emotions and mind.

- Look at your diet. Don't lie to yourself. Change it and start being healthy. It makes a huge difference.
- A dear friend who controls her bipolar disease swears that Omega-3 is an incredibly important and helpful supplement,
- If possible, walk for at least 20–30 minutes each day.
- At least go outside and have a look at a leaf, a flower or a tree. Really examine it. It takes you out of your head.
- Read positive self-help books.
- Make a gratitude list.
- Practise mindfulness!

9

Digest the pain, take the opposite action

Part of our neurotic mind always wants to run, be distracted, avoid. Self-compassion leads to the opposite by enabling us to take the time to face our pain. This is because – as we have already discussed – there is nowhere to run. Unfortunately, we are stuck with our thoughts. Deciding to change them is helpful, applying all the exercises in this book the solution, but while we are in the maelstrom of one neurosis or another, there is only one thing we can do:

Sit with whatever comes up. Instead of trying to avoid it, look at what comes into your mind. Examine its nature. Where is the pain? Where is our anger?

Slowing down and examining what is going on can allow us to make friends with our worst enemy. We can befriend the 'hopeless case' that we are, the ball of anger we become . . . Trying to control our rage or attachment or jealousy is tricky. It's not as if we can put it in our hands. We have to do something that is opposite to how we normally react and use its energy.

If we were to wait for our negative emotions to wear themselves out, we might wait for ever. And pushing them down makes them pop up all the more strongly. Therefore the only solution is taking the opposite action.

Kind and angry thoughts cannot exist at the same time.

We might not be able to rid ourselves of the poison but we can transform it. It's a bit like Jean Valjean in *Les Misérables* turning from the wrong to the right track. We know that indulging whatever negative emotion we harbour does nothing but harm us as well as others. Has acting selfishly brought us happiness? Will getting angry bring us happiness? Will being eaten up with greed bring us happiness?

It is by transforming our anger into love and patience, our jealousy into rejoicing for the other person and our pride into humility, the understanding that we are part of everyone and everything and the dropping of our sense of 'specialness', that will lead to compassion – and to its by-product, happiness.

There's a story of a saint who kept a very angry, grouchy and moody assistant with him at all times. When asked why he did so rather than pick a much better and more suitable candidate, he replied, 'To remind me of why I need to train my mind in compassion.'

I like that quotation because it explains so clearly how we can use our unhappy marriage or difficult colleagues as the perfect fodder to help us to train ourselves out of our misery.

If it isn't pride or anger that prevents our happiness, it can be jealousy. We have looked at pride already, so let us now look at jealousy. Jealousy literally eats away at us. We think the other person has it so much better or easier than us . . . Our partner goes off with a younger model and we would like to kill him. That jealousy makes us lose our dignity and our peace of mind. It robs us of our happiness. We want to lash out, and we start thinking of all the ways we could do so. We invest our minds in imagining all the terrible revenge we could wreak. But would setting his house on fire, flattening his tyres or putting diesel in his petrol tank make us happy? It wouldn't make him happy, but nor would it give us the desired result. Really. We like to think it would, but it wouldn't. After the initial high, it would probably reinforce the sense of our being a 'bad' person and justify our partner's action.

I once saw a fridge magnet that said, 'Happiness is the greatest revenge'.

And another that said, 'Love your enemy, it will drive him crazy'.

I would add another saying, 'Compassion is the greatest strength'.

For the poison of envy is still in our mind and there is no escaping it. Transforming it is best. I personally believe that eating disorders usually have at their root the difficult and hidden emotions of jealousy and envy; along with not feeling good about oneself, and perfectionism.

Rejoice! Rejoice instead.

Eventually mindfulness training can pervade our whole life. That is why meditation, in one particular language, means 'getting used to' . . . We are getting used to our mind being as it really is and training our mind into a way of living whereby we are constantly aware and constantly free, 24 hours a day.

It may be a struggle, but it is one we can win. If we persist in taking the opposite action, the negative emotions will begin to abate and our kindness and compassion will take over.

The habits of negative emotions can attack us, but the power of wanting everyone to be happy and free from suffering means the compassionate wish will eventually triumph against the power of negativity.

Exercise 9

Just before you go to sleep tonight, make the wish that everyone be happy and free from suffering. When you wake up, make the same wish. Keep that same wish on the tip of your tongue for 24 hours and see if you don't feel happier.

Exercise 9a

Make a list of all the people for whom you feel envy or jealousy. Instead of investing your mind in the pain of that poisonous emotion, beam them love. Say quietly to yourself: 'I rejoice that they are together'; 'I rejoice that they have all my money'; 'I rejoice that they are young and healthy' . . . whatever emotion it is that you need to transform.

Exercise 9b

Once upon a time, a beggar appeared before the Buddha, begging for food.

The Buddha looked at him and said: 'I will give you everything you see, all the banquet assembled before your eyes, on one condition. You have to say:

"I have enough."'

The beggar would have said anything, attracted as he was to the beautiful feast before his eyes. So he said, as the Buddha had asked: 'I have enough.'

The Buddha told him to take everything he wanted and off he went quite happily.

The Buddha's students asked him why he had made the beggar do this.

'For hundreds of lives he has been begging and never had enough. By saying "I have enough" he has broken the habit.'

This story is not recounted exactly in its original form but I hope the gist is clear. Now, here is the exercise:

Today get up and say:
'I have enough.'

Simply saying those words stops the sensation that others are all OK and that you don't have enough. It helps you to relax.

10

Anger – why bother?

If the basis of mindful compassion is a calm mind, we cannot afford to have wild emotions. I know many clients who say, 'What would I do without my anger, my emotions? I wouldn't be able to be creative, have fun . . .'

The answer is, try it out. Find out for yourself. The peace you discover on the other side of anger and negative emotion is not comatose but enlivening and happy and compassionate (that word again!).

The damage

This is the chapter that has really made me stall. That is because anger is the emotion about which I have done and still do my most personal research. I have definitely not mastered my own anger yet, so I write from the point of view of a student on the path of training. If any of you out there have heard me angry, I am sorry from the depths of my heart. The good news is that I am well qualified to talk of anger's pitfalls.

As Jigme Khyentse Rinpoche put it quite simply, 'If you give way to your anger completely, you could end up in prison.'

It sounds extreme, but when we glibly 'lose it' on a regular basis, it is as well to be reminded, in much the same way as the increasingly powerful warnings on cigarette packets, that *anger kills*.

Impatience

Some of you might not know what I didn't know for a very long time: anger is often impatience in disguise. Sometimes we think we're angry when actually we are impatient. A client I saw was troubled because he felt he wasn't making progress in resolving his issues. When we looked at his block, it became clear that it was because he was impatient, wanting immediate quick fixes, and he was actually ignoring how much good work he had been doing already.

Chuck Spezzano defines impatience as wanting to get something before it is our time to get it. This can mean we feel guilty when we do get what we want. Because we got it before we were meant to, we don't enjoy it.

If we are always in a hurry, we miss the point. Rushing to a destination means missing the journey. My friend John pointed out that speeding on the motorway doesn't actually get us to our destination that much quicker. Here's the maths:

If you travel at 100 mph instead of 70 mph, you will take 42 minutes rather than 60 minutes to reach your destination – in other words you only lose 18 minutes. Will someone die because you arrive 18 minutes later? Or will someone live because by going 18 minutes slower you haven't run him or her over? Indeed, how many fewer dead insects will you have to clean off your windscreen?

The greatest antidote to anger and impatience is patience!

'In the practice of tolerance, one's enemy is the best teacher,' says the Dalai Lama.

Does that not make sense of our anger more than the anger itself? *If anger meets anger it makes for a greater disaster.*

The joy is in learning that anger, like any other emotion, is a response to a given situation and always serves a purpose. It serves to divide, to make our problem more important than the solution, to get our so-called voice heard. Sometimes it makes us hide away and isolate ourselves; it can make us do anything it wants us to do other than be compassionate.

It is another kick, another high to give us an important sense of ego rather than stay calm.

I remember having an honoured guest to stay. As I showed him around my beautiful city, I told him how angry a particular building made me feel because of the way people within it had treated my young children. I felt strongly justified in being angry, and came out with the usual, 'How *could* they behave in such a way?'

I admitted to him that I was angry, although it was pretty obvious. Even though the event had happened several months earlier, I was still carrying it with me. He looked at me and laughed, saying, 'Why bother?'

To quote Chuck Spezzano again: 'All problems have at root a grievance', or, 'Emotions are complaints that somebody is not doing it your way.'

Beyond the grievance is a greater gift. Always.

When we are angry, we can't see straight and we make rash interpretations and associations. The angry mind can never be happy, so for our own sake as well as those around us, we need to understand our anger and learn to let it go.

If we've never been taught how to deal with anger, either we tend to swallow it until we can't take it any more and so blow our top, or we get an adrenalin rush from the emotional explosion and hope the explosion will mean we get our way, at least in the short term. Bear in mind too that the rush we get from anger can be addictive.

When we lose it, we are more likely to say and do things that we later regret. There's a very popular expression among therapists, 'Own your own emotion.' If we have the self-compassion to realize it is we who are boiling up with anger because of what we feel about something or someone outside us, then we can empower ourselves to express that feeling rather than letting rip.

I have found these three lines among the most helpful for myself and others when trying to deal with anger:

- 'You saying that makes me feel . . .'
- 'You not saying that makes me feel . . .'
- 'You acting that way makes me feel . . .'

Otherwise, as touched on in Chapter 8, we can become so firmly locked inside ourselves that we lose much of our self-esteem, so that it becomes safer and easier to be mad at ourselves than at someone else. This can lead to constant disappointment and greater depression.

Passive aggression

How often have we gone around saying 'I'm fine', when clearly we're not? If smoke really could be seen coming out of our ears, it would . . .

If you grew up in a dysfunctional household, you might not think anger can be expressed in a controlled and healthy way. This is not the case.

Communication and dialogue heals all problems.

Otherwise you can end up subtly encouraging others to take advantage and stop them changing their behaviour. If you've got white knuckles, how can other people know you've been hurt? You stay stuck in the hurt and sense of failure.

Cynicism

It is also worth mentioning cynicism. This is a nasty side of anger. Avoid it at all costs and invest your mind in positive thinking!

'Holding onto anger is like drinking poison and expecting the other person to die.'

The Buddha

From a psychological point of view, anger is most often about control. As described above, we get caught in feeling justified in being angry. We use the emotional manipulation of aggression and then withdrawal. To quote from Chuck Spezzano again:

> At a subconscious level, you have chosen for a person or situation to be the way they are because it allows you to express your buried anger. Anger begins with fear: it is an attempt of one part of your mind to control another. Become aware of your inner conflict and heal it. *Communicate without attacking because attacking stops communication* and does nothing to help your emotional maturity: anger is the adult equivalent of a tantrum. Anger is counterproductive because in trying to control another, it breeds only power struggles as we resort to fight or flight.
>
> TAKE RESPONSIBILITY for the situation that brought about the anger. What have you buried? Bring these elements into the light so you can respond maturely with your conscious mind.

Here are some exercises for transforming anger. Remember:

> 'Our sorrows and wounds are healed only with compassion.'

Exercise 10

If you feel like sounding off, count to ten.

Choosing to do this is vital. Most often we choose not to.

Therefore make the thought of being compassionate greater than that of 'losing it'.

Exercise 10a

When you feel angry, leave the room.

The very act of changing place can dispel the angry emotion.

Exercise 10b

BREATHE AND WAIT.

Research has shown that the neurological anger response lasts less than two seconds.

Exercise 10c

If you stay angry for more than those two seconds, it is because you have a commitment to or investment in staying angry.

Wait and if you are still angry, try this:

Breathe in and out deeply, three times.

Call in your high power, your good heart, and ask profoundly for help.

Despite the situation in front of you, ask yourself when you first felt angry like this. (For the sake of argument, let us randomly say 'at the age of five'.) Know that the first answer that comes to you is always the right one, however obscure it might seem. I have no doubt that the anger you feel right now is a repeat of an earlier situation.

Breathe in and out again.

Ask yourself what was happening to you at the age of five. Give the first answer that pops into your mind.

Let the answer come in. See/feel the situation. What was going on? Who was around? Where were you?

Ask yourself whether you were angry at your father, your mother, God or authority in any shape or form. Answer the first thing that comes into your mind. Sometimes a sibling will pop into your mind as the root of your anger.

Most often the answer is clear and surprising. If it isn't clear, trust that you are avoiding the truth and start the procedure again. Trust the process.

Place a ball of brilliant rainbow light above your head, much like the disc of a full moon. See a line of light connect it to your heart centre wherever you are reading this.

Go to the young person you were at whatever age you picked. See that little you looking angry and distressed. Feel love for her or him.

See a ball of light in that younger you, in the younger you's heart centre. See it connecting to the ball of light above your head. Feel that younger you reconnecting to the interdependent you rather than isolating you in your tantrum, fear or anger.

Let a line of light go from your heart centre wherever you are reading this to the younger you's heart centre, like the lower line of a triangle.

Feel the triangle connecting you wherever you are now in your heart centre to the little you and his or her heart centre and the ball of light above your head.

Feel the light circulating between you and everything else.

Do this until you feel that the original anger or feeling of separation has dissolved.

If you doubt the efficacy of this process, apply faith. Avoid being cynical, as suggested above. Trust that the process has been used thousands of times, achieving huge success and relief. So many people have so many stories of letting go of huge chunks of unexpressed anger, pain or sadness, and of feeling gratitude and relief as a result. Just because it's so easy, don't doubt its power. It helps dissolve blocks that have set you up against the world. Be compassionate with yourself. Use it.

Believe it or not, I have just done it myself again to make sure I had written it down in a comprehensible way. I went back to the age of three, when I remember my older brother pushing me off a brick wall. I had remembered the event before but I had failed to let go of the anger: not only anger at him but anger at my parents, who were busy arguing inside and had failed to see what was happening. I just let go.

Keep on using this exercise if you still feel angry. Maybe there is an even earlier event when you disconnected. Reconnect.

And should you dislike using the white light, imagine giving yourself a hug.

Exercise 10d

If your anger is self-directed, make a list of your positive qualities.

Exercise 10e

However bad your situation, if others can forgive, so can you.

You don't need to take revenge. The law of cause and effect takes account of that. What goes around comes around. Let the universe sort it out rather than trying to do it yourself.

Simply say: 'I forgive'.

Feeling reluctance is understandable, but think how you can now be free and set your family and those around you free.

Lie to yourself, encourage yourself, say it over and over to yourself, until one day, however much further down the line, you will be able to forgive. Or put your heart into it and do it fully right now. There's no time like the present.

Caution: I am not advising meeting with your 'enemy'. I am recommending you do this in the safety of your own home until you feel at peace. What matters is that you dissolve your inner enemy and regain your full heart.

11

Clinging versus loving kindness and compassion

Most of us start out with dreams. Generally, we want a happy life and a good job or a degree. We want to find the ideal partner (yes, I know there are some who want to remain alone) . . . and we want good health.

In the main, we start out wanting to love and have a happy family, and to get things right where according to our perception our parents failed us and went wrong. The problem is that often we navigate our life with unhealed wounds and limited vision. I describe it as floating forwards in our beautiful, dream wedding-gown, but with tins and ropes and junk holding us and pulling us back.

We might have grandiose ideas about being compassionate and loving at all times to friends, family, our new love or new boss. Then, bang, crash, wallop, we fall into the booby trap of what we call love but is actually dependence, neediness, attachment . . . clinging – whatever you might like to call that particular emotion.

I am sure you all know someone who never learnt to drive so their partner would have to drive them around? Or those who say: 'I love you, I love you, I love you' because they need love so badly and can't imagine life without their partner.

Or someone who has hit the bottle because his partner has died after 30 years of marriage and he simply can't let go of her memory and begin to live without her?

Or do you still talk to your children on the phone several times a day even when they have left home and are trying to lead independent lives and are too polite to ask you to give them more space?

Or maybe you are trying to be kind and loving but have an inner voice chattering away about your partner's faults, while you secretly obsess about someone else?

If your wish is 100 per cent for others' happiness at all times, that is fantastic . . . keep going! But most often our needs and attachments and habits and unhealed wounds interfere with love . . .

I asked one of my sons if he had anything clever and quick to say about clinging and he replied, remembering a talk he had been to, 'It's like trying to grab a handful of water in your hands.'

Have you ever tried to do that? It's the same with our thoughts, habits and love . . . little things . . . I moved a plant that had been in the same place in my garden for over 20 years. It still upsets me several days later not to find it where it should be.

Habits. Wanting to keep things the same. Wanting to possess. Wanting things to be permanent.

My son also mentioned the practice of making sand mandalas. The artists spend so much time, effort and attention creating the most wonderful mandalas out of sand, only to destroy them when the work is complete. My own brother used to paint on canvas, and when he wanted to create a new work he would paint over what he had previously done. I admired him as it was so contrary to many artists' wish to show their work, to keep and preserve it.

It's the idea that things are solid and are going to stay solid, and that they will always be there for us, that causes the trouble.

The pain comes from grasping or clinging to something when it is over or when it is not going to happen. We may try and hang on to an event when it has gone, or hang on to a person to fulfil our unmet needs. We think hanging on will give us what we need, whereas it has the opposite effect. Letting go will actually lead to more happiness and space for compassion. For wanting things our own way, or wanting something back the way it was, or wanting another person, place or situation to give us what we are lacking, leads only to attachment and pain. The more attached we are, the more helpless we become. Attachment is like an addiction: it is need disguised as love and means that, for example, we use a partner as a drug. Fantasies are needs too. As we let go of the fantasy, we get back bonding and a real relationship.

Of course we *want* the thing or the person back. We don't want to believe they might be better with someone else. We don't want to indulge in the real love of letting them go.

Choosing – that word again – to unstick is key.

Choosing to be free of clinging is the key to freedom and compassion, both for yourself and others.

Emotional courage is a great thing. Taking responsibility for your emotions is a mature response that will lead to more truth and compassion in your life and the lives of those around you.

As with all things, the more you take responsibility and witness where you are going wrong, the more successful you can be in maintaining calm while ridding yourself of this fake dependence.

Here's an exercise to help you get through this.

Exercise 11

Ask yourself, when did you first feel needy?

Let us say at the age of four.

See the four year old in front of you.

Send love to your four-year-old self.

Wash your four-year-old self through with light.

Hug him or her as you would a needy child. Give yourself all the love you did not receive.

Don't stop until the younger you feels full of love, no longer 'hungry' but full up.

Exercise 11a

Take a deep breath in and out.

Call in the help of your good heart.

Ask yourself how much, on a scale of 1 to 100 per cent, of your mother's or father's pain you swallowed.

Was it 100 per cent? Fifty?

Not burning that pain away creates confusion and lost boundaries.

Ask yourself, if it didn't have all the pain you swallowed in it, what would your life be like?

Ask yourself how it would be if you trusted your good heart instead of trying to deal with it by yourself, as you have been doing since swallowing all the pain.

Ask yourself, how much of your family values did you swallow?

Ask yourself, how much of your parents' example as a couple did you swallow?

Ask yourself if you would be willing to let go and be happy. Really?

Would you really be willing to let go of control and be as light as a bubble?

Then let it all go and hand it back to that 'stuff' beyond your ego. Let interdependence, your high power or your good heart, God, Buddha or Allah handle it.

When you're in pain it's always about the self, and it's caused by our emotions. When you're in trouble, realize it's because you're thinking about yourself. *Take responsibility* for that. If you abstain from negative emotions, you will have constant happiness and be infinitely kinder to others.

Exercise 11b

When you feel obsessed with someone, see him or her as skin and bones and blood, and remember that is what he or she is really made of! Not sugar and spice and all things nice.

Exercise 11c

Remember to apply loving kindness to yourself and to whatever you are attached to.

Then apply loving kindness to everyone, since we are all part of the same team.

Everyone and everything is equal.

Love unconditionally: it transmutes selfish attachment.

Beam that love out impartially to all. It's much better than staying stuck in the attachment.

Exercise 11d

Give whatever it is you are not receiving.

Part 2

The solutions

12

Calm abiding meditation

People charge an awful lot of money nowadays to introduce you to mindfulness, but this information has been available for millennia for free. There is no need to pay vast amounts for it, or indeed to get a few more letters after your name studying it.

It's simply about doing it. Because you pay for it does not mean it is best. *All that glitters is not gold.*

Mindfulness is one of the simplest things in the world to practise. However, as someone said, 'It is simple but not easy.'

This is true. But you could look at it the other way around. Think of it as a challenge. It is a challenge to keep on improving your mind. It is something you need never get bored with because there is always room for improvement. Until you can completely let go and be 100 per cent calm at all times, there is always something to develop while at the same time being happy with where you are, right now.

Maybe this is why so many people who have seen it all and done it all take up the practice with alacrity. Everything else has reached capacity – many challenges have been accomplished. So what next?

Applying the practices that truly lead to freedom from suffering? Yes!

If an analysis were made of the many so-called successful people who have remained on retreat and continued to practise, I reckon a high percentage of them would be personalities who were very successful in business, sport and the media. This is because in spite of their material success they have realized they were bored and often unhappy.

So many of us fail to realize what will truly make us happy and continue to indulge in things that cause us suffering. Applying compassion to oneself is applying tried and tested methods known to alleviate suffering.

Calm abiding meditation is perhaps the most important method of all.

How well have you been doing without training your mind? Do you by any chance spend a lot of time doing other kinds of training? Exercise, sport, sex?

Of course, I am not about to tell you not to do any of those things. But what result do they produce? All those hours training for Wimbledon, and then what?

Training your mind will lead you to freedom.

We are always chasing after what we haven't got and trying to get rid of what we have got. We are constantly fighting this inner battle. Meditation is the road to freedom. There will always be both happiness and unhappiness in life, but mind training ultimately leads you not to be troubled by either. And the by-product is, of course, happiness – but happiness that does not have an opposite. It is a state. It is like taking medicine. As I said before, you can't tell which bit of the course of antibiotics is effective, but you know that overall you feel better. Don't expect immediate results. Don't condemn it if you think one day is dreadful and another good.

Keep at it. And at the end of a year, take a look and if you feel so much as a glimmer of improvement in your well-being, keep going.

This is, after all, for the doubters among you, evidence based. But we need to cultivate it.

Exercise 12

Here is a foolproof method of meditation taught to me by some of the best teachers in the world:

Find a comfortable place to sit. If you can sit cross-legged on a cushion, that is fantastic. If not, sit on a chair. What is important is that your back is straight – not rigid, but following the natural curve of the spine.

Keep your chin fractionally forward and in direct alignment with your spine, and your stomach slightly pulled in. Put your tongue behind your two top front teeth and keep your mouth open just a little, as if you had a grain of rice between your lips.

Relax your shoulders, place your hands loosely on or towards your knees.

Keep your eyes open, gazing upwards if you need to make yourself more alert or downwards if you need to calm your thoughts.

Your posture should be similar to that of a tiger about to pounce, alert but not rigid; or as if you were a mountain, which is naturally inspiring without straining to be so.

Let your mind settle in the same way that mud settles at the bottom of a pond when you leave it unstirred. Watch your monkey mind, watch your thoughts. When you get caught up in your thoughts and become aware you're caught up in them, focus instead on your breathing.

Breathe in and breathe out. Don't breathe in a special way, just normally. If you like, count the breath in as 'one' and count the breath out as 'two'. Don't go beyond two.

No doubt your thoughts will wander, leading you to worry about things you have or haven't done in the past or about things that haven't yet happened. Again, when you find yourself getting caught up in your 'cloud', come back and focus on your breath again.

Don't judge yourself or think you are failing.

Slowly but surely you will mind the gap more and more. Slowly but surely you will begin to perceive the sky-like nature of your mind rather than the distractions.

13

The practice of compassion

As I said earlier on, the practice of compassion has been shown to increase happiness. Studies show, for example, that the frontal lobe of the brain grows as a result of developing compassion. Now we are going to move from resistance to application.

In tests, one set of people were asked to do what they enjoyed most – going to the theatre, swimming, needlework, whatever – and another were asked to do charity work. It was those who did the charity work who scored higher on the happiness scale.

It follows that compassion is the most selfish thing we can do for ourselves.

To repeat, we are talking about the science of the mind – which, incidentally, is the definition of mysticism. It's cutting-edge stuff, and more interesting evidence will emerge as scientists catch up with the greatest computer of all time: our own minds. But then again, does science need to?

It would be helpful now to 'Ride the horse in the direction it is going' instead of persisting in trying to tame our unhelpful bucking broncos. Ignore any remaining voice that resists doing what is helpful. Never mind if your mother told you it was silly, or friends call it 'sissy', or workmates think it 'bizarre'.

Training in compassion doesn't mean we end up being 'high' or happy all the time. That would raise our expectations so much that it would make falling short all the more painful. Training in compassion helps us to develop a baseline, and that baseline grows stronger and stronger until it becomes a way of being. That way of being is the satisfaction derived from 'a good life'.

I don't think there's a person on earth who has led a compassionate life and regretted it. It is a winning way of being, with no possibility of losing. Eventually, as a bonus, it will give us a more accurate understanding of reality.

It is not that suffering will no longer happen, nor that pain is ever desirable. But seeing others' suffering, looking beyond our own concerns, and increasing our awareness of others and our ability to help them, leads to inner peace that is no more affected by happiness than it would be by sadness.

Slowly but surely we can develop a warmer heart and more kindness. And here is a practical way to do so. If you think you have mastered this practice, think again. There was someone who practised nothing but this for over 40 years. Nevertheless, try the following exercise.

Exercise 13: The practice of exchange

Imagine someone you know standing in front of you. See what they look like, what clothes they are wearing, whether they are fat or thin, tall or short, or have brown or purple hair.

Go a little deeper and imagine what it might feel like to be that person with their own issues.

Whenever your mind wanders, bring it back.

Keep going. Try to see things from the other person's perspective. Imagine being in that person's own skin rather than yours. Imagine having that person's problems and not yours.

As the wall between yourself and the other person begins to break down, reverse the usual order and start to breathe in their pain. Visualize it as black smoke.

Now begin breathing out white light onto the person. Imagine light with the consistency of a rainbow but the brilliance of a full moon.

Don't worry if you can't see the smoke or light. If you can, fantastic; if you can't, no trouble. Just keep on breathing in the pain of the other person and breathing out the light.

Whenever your mind wanders, simply come back and carry on.

When you've focused on that particular person for a few minutes, move on to someone else you feel inspired to do it for: your great-grandmother, your great-grandson, your best friend, your worst enemy, your first pet dog, the ant you trod on, whoever pops into your mind. Just keep on breathing in their pain and breathing out the light.

Finally, let your mind settle.

It is wonderful to do this sitting down in a quiet room on your own for a good 20 minutes twice a day, as well as another 20 minutes for the calm abiding meditation. It can also be used anywhere and at any time, for example when visiting sick relatives in hospital, or passing a car accident.

14

The white light visualization

This visualization is not new. Like the techniques I mentioned in the last two chapters, it has been around for millennia. It is simply that many of us have been unaware of these mindfulness practices for a very long time. For the last few hundred years, we have been caught up in a mechanistic view of reality, in the material world. With industrialization we came to believe we were in charge of nature instead of realizing we were part of it.

Until recently, it was hard to access the information needed to learn these practices. We are so very lucky now to have everything at hand and easy to download at the touch of a finger. It could be seen as a second Renaissance, enabling us to remember helpful methods we once knew and have since forgotten. I myself have performed a version of this visualization over 200,000 times, because it works. It purifies. It helps to clear those clouds.

This visualization has helped many people suffering from deep anxiety to sleep at night. I once called a former patient who happened to be in hospital. He had overdosed on cocaine and had a psychotic episode. He said remembering the visualization saved his life . . . although I do hope you don't need to find out its benefit in such a dramatic way.

You don't need to use the visualization in the elaborate form I give it here on each and every occasion. If ever you are afraid, use it then.

If ever you feel tired, pour it over you. If ever you feel like doing it for someone else, send him or her light. It's worth a try, and it's infinitely better than staying in negativity and anxiety.

Before you start:

- don't worry if you don't actually see what you are visualizing. Thinking it is great;
- if you have a problem with thinking about something else, don't panic, just notice you have a block and think about it later,
- if two suggestions come to mind, use one now and another on a later occasion;
- if you prefer, you can download the visualization from my website, <www.carolinelatham.co.uk>

Exercise 14: The white light visualization

Sit or lie down comfortably with your eyes closed and let your body relax.

Imagine a ball of brilliant white light above your head: it is made of rainbow light, not solid but of a beautiful translucent quality. See it shining brightly. In fact it shines so brightly it makes you want to climb into it and sit yourself down.

You're entering it alone but you can take a comfortable chair with you or, if you prefer, mould the earth to fit you. Just make sure you are sitting comfortably.

When you're settled, I would like you to breathe in as deeply as you can and release your breath with a noisy sigh.

Now, I would like you to think of what for you would be the perfect natural scene: the sun, the sea and the sky, or whatever for you is the perfect view. I would like you to see it from the top of the sky to the ground . . .

And then I would like you to expand the view both to the left and the right, and to imagine that you have eyes in the back of your head and can see a full 360 degrees. When you have that full view, please breathe in deeply again, releasing your breath with a noisy sigh.

Next, I would like you to imagine your favourite smell – Chanel

No. 5 or lily of the valley, whatever for you is your favourite smell – and put that in the ball of light.

Then I would like you to imagine your favourite (healthy) taste – a perfectly ripe mango from Pakistan or a juicy Wimbledon strawberry – and put that in the ball of light.

Now I would like you to imagine the perfect sound: Beethoven's Ninth, trickling water, whatever for you is that perfect sound. Put that in the ball of light.

And then I would like you to imagine the perfect touch – a baby's bottom, a piece of moss – and put that in the ball of light.

So in the ball of light you have the perfect sight, smell, taste, sound and touch. When you have them all, I would like you to breathe in as deeply as you can and release your breath.

All that is missing now is the perfect feeling. So I would like you to go back to some perfect moment – maybe the first time you swam in the sea or the time you won a three-legged race at school. Your cheeks were probably bright red, and you felt completely carefree. I would like you to put that energy into the ball of light.

Then I would like you to recall the moment when you first fell in love, that crazy heady feeling when all the lyrics in all the songs were written specially for you and you really could have danced all night and thought that feeling would last for ever. I would like you to put that feeling of 'aliveness' into the ball of light.

Sadly those feelings don't last. But what does last is this ball of light: your perfect space, your safe refuge. It will never run out on you.

Now I would like you to imagine an opening in the crown of your head the width of the stem of a flower, leading from the crown of your head to the ball of light.

From the ball of light a drop of light plops into the inside of your head, and then another drop, until as if pouring from the perfect teapot a steady stream of rainbow white light fills up the inside of your head. Imagine it pouring through your throat, chest, heart, lungs, stomach and intestines, reproductive organs, down both your legs through to your feet.

Beneath you the earth cracks open and out from the soles of your feet pours your pain – physical, mental, emotional or spiritual – into the ground like black oil or manure.

Again, see the light pouring through you, through your head, down the back of your neck, through your spine, across each and every vertebra, down through to your coccyx, down the back of your legs, pushing your pain down and out into the ground as black oil.

And again, the light cascading through you like a powerful waterfall, forcing you to let go of the blocks you quite like hanging on to, pouring through you and dislodging even the most stubborn resistance. Feel it pouring through you, every atom and subatomic particle of your body. Feel it purifying all negativity. Feel it pushing down and out all your negative self-beliefs, all your anxiety, which pour into the ground as black oil or manure.

And one last time, really see the light flowing through you and pushing out any dregs into the ground. Imagine the earth sucking up the last of your pain as if it were the most powerful aspirator in the world. See it close up. Thank it for taking your pain.

You are now left in nothing but light. From there I would like you to send that light to one other significant person in your world.

Feel yourself a little like someone on the moon . . .

15

Compassion towards oneself

In Ladakh, in the Himalayas, until a generation or so ago, people lived in community. If two people married, both sides of the family would come together and build the newlyweds a house. Everything was shared and recycled. This sense of interdependence and value was innate. The couple would receive the gift from the community as members of their community, and no doubt would do the same for the next couple to marry.

In general, this is the exact opposite of our experience in the West, and increasingly in the Middle East. From early on in their lives, people experience isolation, self-hatred and lack of confidence. We touched on this in Chapter 8.

In the course of writing this book I have become aware of the psychological research on self-compassion done by Kristin Neff and Paul Gilbert. Both experts in the field, they confirm how important it is to apply self-compassion, particularly in cases of repeated abuse and violence.

We could go into a definition of 'self', but this might become complicated and not serve the purpose of this book. I like the way Matthieu Ricard puts it. He suggests we should ask ourselves, 'What is really helpful for me?'

'To avoid pain' might be a pretty good reply.

Somewhere along the line we seem to have lost or to have become confused about what it really means to be compassionate to our-selves. We might also have become confused about what is really good or helpful for us. And some of us have known compassion towards ourselves only very little, if at all.

For example, if you have five kids and you give to them so much that you never relax, rest or get enough sleep, you are in danger of eventually cracking up. Of course, you want to put your children first, but it is essential to look after yourself so you can look after them. That's self-compassion. If you don't take time to eat and you end up fainting, it's not going to help anyone.

If you don't show compassion towards yourself, you can end up extremely unhappy and bitter and without love. A workaholic running a company might be looking after his hundreds of staff, but if he is not looking after himself because he is working so hard, he can end up miserable, or with compromised health.

This raises the question of how to apply compassion towards oneself without becoming selfish. So let's look at the difference between self-compassion and something it's often confused with, self-esteem.

Some people take up self-esteem classes with great enthusiasm and afterwards go round selling themselves to themselves as well as to all those around them. They are people who have learnt, as I did, to 'smile when you dial'.

This is because people relying on external self-esteem have to live up to their own standards of perfection and often feel they are falling short of those standards, or whatever they imagine to be expected of them. That can lead to depression, constantly failing expectations and a sore jaw from the plastic smile on your face.

Perhaps the difference can be best explained by a poem I men-tioned in my first book. It's a fable by La Fontaine and it's called 'The Oak and the Reed'. I tried to think of another example, but it seems to me that La Fontaine said it all most clearly 500 years ago. The gist of the poem is this:

The oak is very proud and boasts to the reed about how powerful he is.

'Look at me, I'm big and strong. You're so small and puny and you should emulate me . . .'

The reed is humble and thanks the oak, looking up admiringly at the big, loud, noisy tree . . .

At that very moment, a huge storm comes along and fells the oak tree in two – dead.

The little humble reed has bent over in the wind and comes out unscathed.

I like to explain the reed's bending in the wind as being 'naked'. If you are indulging in pride borne of self-esteem, you can be felled. If you are 'naked' and know that you are part of everything, then you cannot disconnect from that truth and are 'nakedly loving'.

You aren't wearing a suit. You aren't hiding behind your profession. You aren't torturing yourself by trying to keep up a front. You're not presenting a label. You are yourself.

You love yourself as you did when you were a baby. Of course there are tragic exceptions, but in most cases babies naturally love themselves. They are oblivious to the idea of guilt. They are oblivious to having to play a game or the need to perform. They are oblivious to the idea of needing a prop.

They smile and it is as if they were naturally meditating when at rest . . . Nor do they lack compassion towards themselves when they want food or a cuddle.

They make themselves heard and ask for their needs to be met.

People often seem to think that becoming compassionate or growing to be a good person is something way out there, unattainable, over the rainbow.

Yet it is not so. It is learning to undo the mistaken beliefs we have developed along the way, returning to our natural 'baby' self and our natural way of feeling compassion towards ourselves before the rot set in. But the rot can be removed. That is the journey of self-compassion: to clear out the mistaken jumble, the rot and clutter.

There's another simple method of developing self-compassion: by not doing harm.

Harming either others or oneself is the opposite of compassion.

It's that simple, but we will always try and complicate things.

How often have you rewarded yourself with a packet of chocolate biscuits, or a drink, or chips, and thought you were being good to yourself? Yet if you are 'good to yourself' in that way every day, the weight will pile on and the effect will be far from self-compassionate.

Actions have reactions, so it is important to consider what compassion to yourself really is and not to cheat or be in denial . . .

To avoid harming yourself means to take the actions that will lead to your happiness. Since we know that happiness is borne of compassion, every action you do to benefit others will be one of self-compassion. And every action you do that is genuinely helpful to yourself will be an act of self-compassion too.

If you don't take care of yourself, you cannot take care of others. If you're on the scrapheap, you're not going to be much good to anyone else.

Sacrifice

Try to avoid insidious sacrifice. Sacrifice is compassion's false friend and allows you to go without so that you can score points off giving to the other person. It is not free giving.

It leads you to think: 'I'm so great because I've suffered so much today doing all the work you laid around.' It seeks praise. It often seeks to hold partners or children hostage. 'You owe me because I did all that for you.'

It is where you give but do not receive and fear of intimacy and success may lead you to hide in 'the job', in the 'doing'. You may be trying to prove you are good enough because you don't actually believe it. The awareness born of mindfulness can help us to see how we act and whether it is with or without an agenda. It helps us to see our patterns of behaviour and begin to avoid their pitfalls. It helps us test our motivation.

It helps us to ensure that our motivation is always to benefit others as much as possible.

Exercise 15: Think before you act

Before you take any action that may affect others, ask yourself: will this action lead to happiness or to more unhappiness?

Take the action that will be of most benefit to others while not doing harm to yourself.

Exercise 15a: Seeking innocence

Sit down quietly.

Breathe in deeply and breathe out deeply.

Call in your good heart to access your unconscious.

Sit until you feel present and aware of your body as you sit.

When you are fully present, ask yourself this:

On a scale of 0 to 100 per cent, how much have you lost of the innocence you had as a baby who felt full compassion for himself or herself? (Apologies if you were one of those who had a terrible start to life!)

Take the first answer that comes into your mind as true.

For the sake of simplicity, let's say the answer is 40 per cent.

Now, take another deep breath in and out.

Call in your good heart again.

Ask yourself at what age you lost that innocence.

Let the answer come in.

Let's say it was four.

See in front of you the four year old who has lost her or his innocence and is operating only at 60 per cent. There are multifarious reasons why this could be: a parent leaving or dying, parental criticism, an accident, bullying by a sibling, going to nursery. It could be anything . . . anything that would have sent you off balance and stopped you trusting that you were 100 per cent loveable.

See opposite you the 60 per cent of you that knows you are innocent and fully loveable.

Step forward and hug her or him until you merge and are 100 per cent innocent and 100 per cent valuable again.

Cry those tears, since they are real tears rather than crocodile tears. Just feel the sadness as long as it lasts. It will end and you will feel better.

If you didn't pick an age and you have never felt innocent, either you are not being honest with yourself, or you are trying too hard – although on some rare occasions, it could be because your mother went through a traumatic pregnancy. If so, imagine yourself in the womb and do the same exercise again.

If you couldn't do it, don't think you have failed. Just start again tomorrow and trust it will work and will help.

16

Compassion for family

As we have now become aware, we have built up our ego from early in childhood in order to learn to cope with life and to become functional, rational adults. But that ego may have become warped to compensate for our unmet childhood needs and to cover up our pain.

Whatever happens to us in life can have a positive, negative or neutral effect, and we can respond to anything and everything in a positive, negative or neutral way. But *family* definitely incites strong reactions in most of us, while parents often incite even stronger reactions.

There are those who have a particular bias: 'Of course I'll do that for my family but not for anyone else. I love my family so much.' More often – or maybe that's just a therapist's experience – one hears the opposite reaction: 'Of course I'll do that for anyone but I won't go near my family.' Or, 'Leave me alone and don't mention my family or my parents. I don't want to know.'

Taking the trouble to look at these responses and go beyond their limitations, bothering to do a compassionate exercise or two, might help release some of this angst and allow us to develop more freedom to love. Instead of maintaining reserve and keeping our distance, we could release our pain into happiness and compassion. As a very dear friend of mine in Canada said at the end of a course we had done together, 'I knew I was in hell, but I forgot I could let myself out of it.'

We tend to blame much of our lack of love, unhappiness and insecurities on our parents. Most often we blame them, as Larkin's poem puts it so politely, for getting it wrong. There are always exceptions to the rule but we are speaking of the generality. We tend to blame them for many of our shortcomings or pain and then we catch the same problem and transfer it onto our children. If we don't blame them, we blame ourselves.

If we don't look at the pain, we tend to carry it unconsciously around with us. We all react and respond differently, but most often there is a lot of residual pain hidden within us long after we have left the roost. What we don't heal we tend to repeat, and it limits our compassion and our behaviour. It will also limit our children's behaviour because they follow our example. For example, so many children grow up to do exactly the same job as their parents did and never learn how to go beyond their parents' limitations.

The ultimate bargaining tool in therapy is that any progress you make in sorting yourself out will be handed down to your children. Even if you don't have children, you are still short-changing yourself and the world if you fail.

Helping to heal some of the problems we have inherited from our parents can save struggle and time. While we are busy training our minds with mindful compassion, the exercises in this chapter can help boost our clarity and give us a kick-start. They are aids, like a first aid kit for temporary repairs to gashes in the mind.

We have a choice. Either we catch our parents' unhelpful behaviour and go on to repeat it, or we look at the behaviour, dump the junk, and bring in the wisdom we can offer both our parents and ourselves.

By that, I don't mean that we can do away with our past. We cannot change where and how we were born and into which family. What we can do is re-address the present.

Now you are an adult, you do not have to react to other adults like a child. *You can learn to respond as an adult to an adult.* When a therapist told me that, it was a lightbulb moment. You no longer have to keep looking up to your parents or following their way of being. You are now free to be equal. That doesn't mean disrespecting them in any way, but it does mean changing the balance. You can become equals.

You don't need to keep on making the same mistake or putting up with the same problem. You can move beyond.

I have seen so many people fearful at the thought of one or other parent seeing them change their behaviour or speak to them in a different manner. Let me reply, 'If you speak your truth from the heart, they will respond rather than react and you will both step into more happiness.'

I hope the simple yet effective exercises below will help you as they have helped many others.

Exercise 16: Giving to your parents

Make absolutely sure you are sitting quietly for this exercise. Don't rush it, because it is very precious. If you are in a hurry, put it aside and do it later.

Call in help, and answer the following questions. Go with the first thing that pops into your mind. Don't censor your answers.

> What would have been the quality your parents most needed as a couple? Not as individuals but as a couple. What would have made their marriage work? Or work better? Most often people suggest things like 'compassion', 'forgiveness' or 'more understanding', 'to work less', 'more love' or 'sobriety' – whatever pops into your mind as being the quality that would most benefit them both.
>
> Visualize yourself giving them that quality. You might picture a gold platter and imagine yourself handing the quality to them on the platter. See them receiving it. If you want, hug them and give it to them that way. See them receiving it. See it melting into their heart and thus relieving their problem.

This enables you to get out of the way. Very often, people have made an early decision as a child to do a better job than one or both of their parents because the parents were obviously failing. If this was you, be aware that you were too young at the time to make a mature and wise decision about how to help them out.

It is time now to remove yourself from the equation. It is time right now to let them get on with it. Whether they were in the happiest marriage or locked in the most bitter divorce, that was their decision, their choice. People can make the most horrific decisions, but that is their right. Free will exists.

Next!

Ask yourself now what would be the quality your father most needed and didn't have. How would it be to bring him this quality as a gift, rather than letting him stay stuck in the problem? Or finding yourself stuck with the memory? Again, this gift could be anything: sobriety, honesty, peace, love, compassion. You name it.

Then visualize yourself bringing in that quality. See your father receiving it. Visualize yourself hugging him if that feels right.

Then give yourself the quality. Whatever it is your father lacked, you could probably do with it yourself right now . . .

Next!

Ask yourself now what would be the quality your mother most needed and didn't have. How would it be to bring her the gift of that quality rather than leaving her to stay stuck in the problem? Or you to stay stuck with the memory?

As with your father, the gift could be anything: sobriety, honesty, peace, love, compassion. Again, you need to name it.

Then visualize yourself bringing in that quality. See her receiving it. Hug her too if that feels right.

Then give yourself the quality. Whatever it is your mother lacked, you could do with it yourself right now as well . . .

That's it. This is an amazingly effective way to discover and then own where you have gone out of balance. Please value its power and know all it is doing.

Note: you might also find it helpful to do this exercise with a therapist or a close and trusted friend.

Exercise 16a

If you belong to one of those families where everything was perfect, your parents may still benefit from the exercise above. If, however, there are no burning issues and you love your parents absolutely and unconditionally, then:

Send that love and compassion out to the whole world.
Widen the scope.
Don't let it be partial.
Extend that love to benefit all.
Remember it will benefit you!

Exercise 16b

Practise treating your family as you would anyone outside of your family. We have complex relationships with our nearest and dearest and if we can 'detach' and treat them normally as we would a friend or even stranger, it can make an immense difference.

Exercise 16c

If you are feeling bold and ready to take on a challenge, try this exercise.

If everything is interdependent, it means that everything can be seen as a mirror or a projection of yourself. Using this idea in therapy saves a great deal of time.

When my marriage broke up, I predictably blamed my husband but I reluctantly came to realize that I had subconsciously set up our split because I hadn't fully healed some past family traumas. I had to take responsibility and be willing to forgive him but also forgive myself.

Breathe in and out.
Call in help.
Ask yourself: What do I find wrong in the person I am living with? Think of whoever it is you have issues with.
Let us say it is because that person is angry, or lies so much. Whatever. Make a list.
Imagine the person standing in front of you and ask yourself this:
'What do I believe about myself to invite this person's behaviour?'

or

'How am I so angry, or lying so much? How is this my mirror?'

As the person stands before you, own responsibility for that projection.

Realize that if someone is treating you badly it is because, somewhere in your unconscious, you believe you deserve to be treated badly. (I did say this was a challenge!)

Give up that belief. Be willing to feel your feelings as they come up. Feel them thoroughly.

Then choose another way. Commit to the truth. Let go of that negative belief.

Take a step closer to the person in your mind. It was your belief setting up the mirror.

Repeat this for as long as your list of complaints about the other person exists.

When you have finally dissolved them all, give the person a hug.

That's big stuff. Well done!

17

Compassion for the world

Somebody once said to me – well before the advent of recycling – 'When you start developing compassion, you end up caring about where you put your rubbish.'

As we develop more awareness we become increasingly concerned about what is going on around us. When we throw a cigarette stub on the ground or forget to take our recyclable bag to the supermarket, we might even develop guilt about the harm we are causing. How wonderful! It's not wonderful to hang on to the guilt, but to feel remorse and to make another choice to act with awareness and consideration and compassion would be splendid.

I have one friend who is quite revolutionary in his approach to compassion. It is deeply affecting. He challenges the accepted manners and modes of behaviour with which we were brought up; for example, when in a restaurant, he piles up the plates and *helps* the waiter or waitress. Instead of treating them almost as paid servants, he is the humble one.

Having him to dinner is a novel experience. The meal is kept as simple as possible: instead of buying the best paper napkins and putting out side plates and water and wine glasses, we eat from a single plate and use a single glass. After all, why use several plates that will require more effort to wash them up and more water to clean them? Compassion is simple and common-sense in application, even if it does challenge the mores we have been brought up with.

If he goes to the beach with us, he disappears to pick up every bit of rubbish in sight. His actions are extremely disturbing to the ego.

But his favourite practice is to buy lobsters and crabs and return them to the ocean, and all his friends are doing the same now. Cutting off the string that binds their claws and letting them move about is one of the greatest joys one can experience. Children love it.

In any way he can be, at any given moment, he is of service to others. He often ends up cooking me supper in my own home when he is the honoured guest. I have to watch out because afterwards he will even start sweeping the kitchen floor!

He somehow makes the simplest fare the most tasty you have ever eaten. I still remember the rice and dhal he cooked five years ago in Sydney but can't remember any of the expensive meals I've eaten in restaurants since then. Why is that?

It's because all he does, lives and breathes is imbued with compassionate awareness. It's catching. Not quickly enough, and resistance is strong, but it is catching. Since he travels worldwide, he has a global effect. He treats everyone as if they are his brother or sister, knowing full well that we all have the same nature and are all struggling in our very often lamentable pits of ego.

He treats animals with the same respect as humans. I once found him getting out chairs to put over an ant trail so people wouldn't inadvertently squash them underfoot. I watched a video of a 90-year-old turtle he returned to the ocean seeming to do a 'thank you' dance before disappearing off for good. He also showed me one of a lorry-load of live fish being tipped back into the ocean.

Truly, if we really look at things, we are all living on one small planet and so far it is our only home. Our home is damaged and in need of careful handling. It is selfish and dishonest – and often lazy, sometimes we just can't be bothered – not to handle it carefully. I know this from personal experience.

When we do bother we feel so much better. We develop increasing self-worth and confidence and we lose our fear of others.

The Dalai Lama says:

I believe that at every level of society – familial, tribal, national and international – the key to a happier and more successful world is the growth of compassion. We do not need to become religious, nor do we need to believe in an ideology. All that is necessary is for each of us to develop our good human qualities. I try to treat whoever I meet as an old friend. This gives me a genuine feeling of happiness. It is the practice of compassion.

Exercise 17

Today, resolve to do one of the following as often as you can:

- If you leave your reusable shopping bag in the car, go back to the car to collect it.
- Pick up some rubbish.
- Let a fly out of a closed room.
- Use a single plate for your meal.
- Turn off an unnecessary light.
- Set aside part of your garden to grow organic produce for your family and friends.
- If you don't have a garden, consider getting an allotment.
- Recycle all waste.
- Use less water.
- Walk or cycle whenever possible.
- Get a folding bicycle.
- Join a carshare scheme.
- Eat a little less (mmm . . .).
- Eat meat only once a week.
- Eat more vegetables and ideally become vegetarian.
- Plant a tree.
- Slow down.
- Begin educating yourself on environmental issues.
- Educate your children about what matters in life.
- Don't leave waste on your plate.
- Whatever you eat, drink or wear, do it in a mindful way.

Epilogue

It is with genuine bewilderment that I finish this book. I feel so much gratitude that I have been able to explore the subject in depth. What a wonderful opportunity my editors have afforded me!

I am still very much an independent operator and like to do things my way. What has astounded me is how other people all over the world have drawn the same conclusions and applied many identical methods to the ones I have been using for decades, alone in my therapy room.

Truth will out.

It is a new beginning.

Genghis Khan used to enjoy saying: 'Happiness lies in conquering one's enemies, in driving them in front of oneself . . . and savouring their despair.'

One could not consider him urbane. An editor of the magazine *The Week*, Jeremy O'Grady, suggests: 'The quality of urbanity has got lost in the global village. We have reverted to being peasants.'

We do run this risk, even though we don't indulge in bloody murders at the rate we used to. (In his latest book, *Altruism* (Atlantic Books, 2015), Matthieu Ricard quotes the rate of murder as having drastically diminished.)

While everyone else is busy thinking the world is ending and our degenerative behaviour catastrophic, I think the people who know how to lead us out of the hole we have dug ourselves have appeared here, there and everywhere to do just that. Many pass by unrecognized and shun any form of publicity, but they are having an effect. They are saving our world by showing us as individuals how to save ourselves, and then to take that attitude outwards.

To quote the Dalai Lama again:

All the world's major religions with their emphasis on love, compassion, patience, tolerance and forgiveness can and do promote inner values. But the reality of the world today is that grounding ethics in religion is no longer adequate. This is why I am increasingly convinced that the time has come to find a way of thinking about spirituality and ethics beyond religion altogether.

What I do know is that what is contained within these pages is beyond the description of any church or any label. Compassion is what makes us tick. Compassion, not money, is what makes the world go around. It is not greed or war or stupidity that will make any of us happy. What will is developing compassion.

I hope from the depths of my heart that as many of you as possible will feel able to put these exercises into practice and help transform this world. It is time for a compassionate revolution. Be warriors of the heart! Break down barriers with your compassion! Shock your negativity into compassionate action! Get a kick out of your positive motivation!

Then you can both live and die happy. This is not about being squeaky clean; it's about being in alignment with your mind and its true nature.

What the world needs now is you!

Have a good heart.

And, in the inimitable words of Jigme Khyentse Rinpoche:

'If you've got something kind to say, say it, otherwise shut up!'

Further reading

Jigme Khyentse Rinpoche (www.songtsen.org)
Chuck Spezzano (all books)
The Dalai Lama (all books)
Dzigar Kongtrul Rinpoche (all books)
Matthieu Ricard (all books)